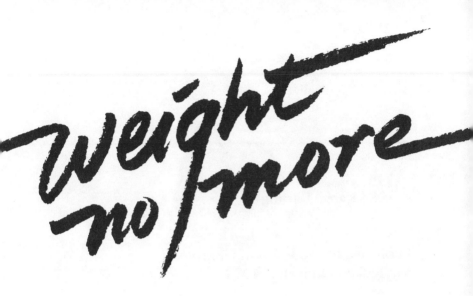

KAREN DARLING

NEW WORLD LIBRARY
SAN RAFAEL, CALIFORNIA

Published by New World Library
San Rafael, California, 1984

Revised and published by Karen Darling 1991

Cover design by Kathleen Vande Kieft
Photo by Christopher Briscoe

Fifth printing 1991

ISBN 0-931432-18-9

DEDICATION

To all my wonderful clients and students, who have taught me so much.

CONTENTS

ACKNOWLEDGEMENTS

Many people deserve acknowledgements for their support in writing this book: most of all, my daughter, Heather. Thank you for your love, support, encouragement, and toleration in listening to my constant talk about "the book."

Deep appreciation goes to Michael Bass and Lorena Laforest Bass for their belief in me; to my dear friend, Jackie Schnitzer, who read, reread, and provided excellent feedback on the manuscript through its various stages; and to my publishers, Jon Bernoff and Mark Allen. You are all wonderful. Mere words fail to express the depths of my gratitude. Many thanks also go to my editor, Carol Conn, whose encouraging phone calls and professional expertise helped me through the final weeks of work on the book.

Being an animal lover, I also want to thank my pet friends: my dogs, Ron and Sarah; my cats, Rita, Abe, and Marilyn. They are always there with unconditional love.

INTRODUCTION

"Please, help me! I want to be thin."

"I want to look like the women in those diet soda ads."

"I want my husband to think I'm beautiful."

These are often the first statements women make when they come to my office for weight counseling.

"Why?" I always ask.

Jaws drop, eyes widen. They look back at me in astonishment. Such a question! Isn't it obvious? They grasp for words, struggling to articulate heartfelt emotions.

My work as a counselor specializing in weight control has given me the opportunity to talk to many women about their bodies. I've listened to their fears and concerns. Many women have unfortunately come to believe that their self-worth is a direct result of how good their bodies look. The bottom line seems to be that they have to be "fashion-model thin" and beautiful to be happy. This is usually what motivates women to get started on crazy, harmful diets.

I feel that the poor self-image so many women have is the logical outcome of our society's placement of women in the role of "sex objects." It's not easy to detach yourself from the cultural obsession with being thin. Turn on the television, pick up a magazine, or listen to the radio: advertisers spend a fortune trying to convince you that being thin will make you rich, beautiful, and happy — especially if you buy their products. It is no simple feat to tune out this onslaught.

I have a basic, practical philosophy about a woman's relationship to her body. I believe her body's size and appearance should be her own concern. It should not be subject to the arbitrary whims of "fashion," which change from year to year. After all, one's body is a highly individual and personal part of one's existence. Being "fashion-model thin" is not bad — if it is your body's natural state. However, it just isn't for everyone.

My goal in this book is to teach you how to be the person *you* want to be, to have the body *you* want, and to eat the way *you* want. This is your God-given right as a human being. You deserve it. And now you can have it.

When you come across the words "slim," "slender," and "thin" throughout this book, please understand that I am referring to how these words relate to you as an individual — not how the fashion magazines and advertisers define them. Do yourself a favor and keep this wise old adage in mind, always: "Beauty is in the eye of the beholder."

As you work through the process of physical and mental change, you might keep the following poem in mind. I found this inspirational gem framed, tucked away in the inner recesses of a garage sale in Denver, Colorado. It contains a valuable lesson and I hope you benefit from it as much as I have.

Up along the way so weary,

When we falter on the trail,

Comes a voice that's kind and cheery,

"Perseverance will not fail."

Then an unseen force impels us,

Stirs the fires of our soul.

And a kindly spirit tells us,

"Cling to hope you'll win the goal."

—Homer S. Nelson

1

GIVE UP DIETS

I tried them all, too. The first was the so-called Mayo Clinic Diet. I'm sure it must have been designed by grapefruit growers. Whenever I eat a grapefruit now, I have to stop and remind myself I am not on a diet.

Then there's the meal you blend up and force down, all the time convincing yourself this is a complete meal and you should be satisfied. But of course, you are not. You are still pining for fried chicken and mashed potatoes.

Remember dragging your scales everywhere, trying to convince the waiter you were conducting scientific re-search as you scooped your portion of fish on the scales platform? And how about all the other gimmicks to which you have surrendered your fragile hopes and your pocketbook?

On my most disgusting list is the plastic suit I wore to bed, naively trying to bid farewell to the fat I was supposed to sweat off during my eight hours of beauty rest. I woke up exhausted, unable to sleep because I was encased in an excrutiating "hot house." And I was still as fat as ever.

Even Webster's dictionary has discouraging things to say about diets. It defines the word "diet" as a "(1) daily food allowance; (2) way of life; and (3) limited food or drink." Doesn't it make your blood boil to have your food "allowance" forever "limited?" And to think of all your past dieting failures as a "way of life?" Sorry, but that's not my idea of living.

Dieting is not a natural way to eat. Dieting is obsessive behavior.

According to American Medical Association statistics, diets have a 95 percent failure rate. I'm not sure how the American Medical Association actually defines dieting success and failure. I define success as *the ability to achieve permanent weight loss without being plagued with thoughts of food, while eating exactly what you want and when you want it and still retaining your perfect weight.*

You will learn how to achieve all these "successes" in this book.

DIETS ARE THE PROBLEM, NOT FOOD

We dieters tend to look upon food as an enemy — A big, bad villain that can get us when our guard is down. It haunts our minds, lurking in the corners wherever we go. Is there no escape from this omnipotent foe?

Actually, it is *the act of dieting* that keeps food in this adversarial position. You know from experience that as soon as you vow to start a diet, you also start thinking about what foods you can and can't have. How many calories are in this? What sacrifices must you make to indulge in it? You become weaker as you face your fifth scoop of cottage cheese and fantasize more about German chocolate cake. This is when the enemy can so easily close in and claim victory once again.

We have to finally recognize that we cannot subject ourselves to diets any longer. We deserve both good food and slender, healthy bodies.

DEPRIVATION DOESN'T WORK

My interest in weight loss means I read a lot of the diet articles in magazines. Often they have titles along the lines of, "Learn to Eat Like a Thin Person." And they usually are variations on the same old theme: food deprivation! That is not how a naturally thin person eats. A naturally thin eater will eat any food she desires with no regard for the caloric content. She never passes up an opportunity to satisfy her desire for apple pie a la mode, which would definitely be on the "no-no" list for a dieter. The thin person, however, eats only enough to satisfy. This is an important point. *Only enough to satisfy.* She doesn't bloat herself.

The dieter eats apple pie with such overwhelming guilt that she has to eat way too much just to numb her feelings of disgust. Consider how a naturally thin eater would react if she were told she had to diet. No more high-calorie foods. Deprive; go without. Chances are her behavior would become like that of the overweight person: she'd start sneaking food, eating when she is not hungry, eating abnormal amounts, thinking of nothing but food. I feel certain she would gain weight for the first time in her life, simply because she abandoned her natural way of eating.

Notice that when I refer to a thin person, I say "naturally thin." This person is very different from the "thin" person who lives on lettuce leaves and carrot sticks, washed down with diet sodas. The naturally thin person eats only quality food. She won't bother with the cardboard-like cookies in the grocery store. She makes sure her cookies are the best.

Dieters, on the other hand, go ahead and stuff down those awful old, stale crackers they found in the camper left over from last summer. They rationalize by telling themselves, "I hate to waste these — they cost $1.79."

A dieter's whole existence revolves around food. She is so preoccupied with thinking about food that she has little time left for creativity, work, pleasure, friends, and above all, her own personal needs. The dieter's first thoughts of the day are usually, "What am I going to struggle not to eat today that would add five more pounds to my thighs?"

What a way to start the day! Where are the positive thoughts that can start your day in the right direction? Lost, submerged, pushed away with thoughts of *food*. By thinking like this, she begins to lose all regard for herself. Her self-esteem is damaged and the possibility of success in all areas of her life is severely undermined.

STOP SETTING YOURSELF UP FOR FAILURE

Diets establish a "failure consciousness." You can probably recall some of your own experiences. Remember standing at the supermarket magazine counter? On the cover of a well-known publication you see the words, "The Only Diet That Works." You frantically grab it off the rack, pay the cashier, race home, and read about this latest "magic" diet declaring, "This is for me! I am really going to succeed with this one. Really!"

This all happens on a Saturday afternoon. You decide to start on Monday. Then you remember the bag of donuts in the kitchen. You promptly walk in and eat them all. You know you have to get rid of them. You don't want them around Monday morning. This pattern of clearing out the goodies for D-day continues throughout the weekend.

D-day arrives. You make it through the first day without cheating. The second day is not quite as good — a little ice cream cone isn't that much, though. By the third day, you can't stand it any longer. Nothing, I mean nothing, is as important as food. You are completely obsessed with it.

Of course, you give in, seriously questioning the sanity of the creators of this diet. You are sure that *he* has always been really skinny and is, for some reason or other, diabolically out to torture all the chubbies of the world. You have managed to justify your defeat on an intellectual level — but subconsciously you are chalking up yet another *failure.* The powerful thought, "I am a failure," starts creeping into other areas of your life. If your subconscious mind believes you are a failure as a dieter, it has the ability to shift that negative belief to your marriage (making you believe you are a failure as a partner), to your job, even to your role as a parent. The subconscious mind does not have the ability to be rational and make judgements; it takes everything literally. So if you believe you are a failure in losing weight, your subconscious mind interprets that to mean you are a failure in general.

Even worse were all the instances in which you managed to stay on a diet for a long time. For *two months* you were a slave to your calorie counter. You turned down invitations to parties or gatherings where a diabolical creme puff might be lurking. Your family was completely fed up with you and your crabby disposition. But you lost 50 pounds!

So you celebrated, by treating yourself to the dieter's reward: a hot fudge sundae. It was such heaven to eat again that you found it impossible to stop there. Little by little, your food intake increased. Within a month you had not only gained back the 50 pounds, but seven more. In your mind, you are the weakest, most disgusting failure existing on the planet. The real tragedy here is that you suffered through the diet hoping to achieve permanent weight loss. In reality you have produced the all-too persistent thought, "I am a failure. I can't do anything right." And you now weigh more than before you started the diet.

YOUR METABOLISM HATES DIETS

Yale University recently released a study indicating diets actually contribute to obesity. The study involved people who had dieted off and on over a long period. It seems when a person goes on a diet, their metabolism (the rate the body burns calories) slows down to meet a diminished intake of food. When the person goes off the diet, their metabolism cannot react quickly enough to meet the greater intake of food. This is why a dieter can lose 10 pounds and then quickly gain 15 after she resumes her normal eating habits. This practice of up-and-down metabolism creates a body unable to regulate itself. The body's natural metabolic process is "confused" and doesn't know how to react.

My theory is that the process of metabolism finally becomes so confused that it says, "I quit — I don't know what you want me to do." And it stays "stuck." I believe this is why I get so many women in my counseling practice who are 45 and older. They have been on diets for so many years they can no longer lose weight.

I have them compile a food chart to determine what they are eating. When I see they are eating like a bird and still can't lose a pound, I tend to believe their metabolism has declared a stand-off. They have to get back to a regular, sensible way of eating, without the on-diet/off-diet cycle. Only then can the body get a clear understanding of what it is supposed to do.

REGAIN YOUR POWER — NOT YOUR POUNDS

The tragic price of dieting is that you give up your personal power. You let something outside of you take care of your needs. If the diet fails, so do you. This leaves you powerless. When you take the matter into your own hands and start to look for those inner reasons you overeat, learning to deal with them in positive ways, you will have given yourself back the power and ability to succeed.

The purpose of this book is to show you exactly how to do just that.

REMINDERS FROM CHAPTER ONE

1. Dieting makes food seem like the enemy. When it is the enemy, you can't relax with it.

2. A naturally thin eater never deprives herself of food, even if it is high in calories.

3. Eat what you want, but only enough to satisfy.

4. Diets establish a "failure consciousness."

5. Dieting can actually contribute to obesity by disregulating your metabolism.

2

THE REASONS
YOU OVEREAT

Food itself has very little to do with being overweight. It is using food to compensate for our unresolved subconscious needs that gets us into weight troubles. We all have our own personal ways to express frustrations, pain, and upsets. Some people turn to alcohol and drugs. A vast majority turn to food.

Frequently my clients will say the reason they are overweight is simply because they love food. This excuse just doesn't hold water. Ask a naturally thin friend if she enjoys good food — chances are very good that she does.

19

The old standby, "I must have a slow metabolism," won't work either. The idea that there are different metabolic speeds (to explain vast weight differences) has no scientific foundation. Nor is it true that your metabolism slows enough to cause inevitable weight gain as you get older. Medical experts conclude the metabolism slows a tiny bit, but not enough to take the blame for that excess 20 pounds. And the "overactive" glands we are sure we must have — only a very small minority can attribute their weight gain to a glandular imbalance.

"Studies show that there is no difference in the way fat and thin people process food in their bodies," states Dr. Edward Marshall, author of *The Marshall Plan.* "The idea that people have different kinds of metabolism — that some people burn up food immediately while others turn it into excess fat — is simply not supported by scientific evidence."

We human beings are complex organisms, however, and many of us have managed to upset our natural balance by weird eating habits, commonly referred to as dieting.

GETTING TO KNOW YOU

There is just no getting around it: food in itself does not pose a physiological problem. But food does have a great *psychological* significance for most of us.

You must understand this significance in order to overcome your weight problem. As you begin to explore your psychological attachment to food, keep in mind you will probably dredge up some painful memories, guilty feelings, and a whole menagerie of other unpleasant beasts. Yet it is essential to be direct and honest with yourself: being honest will pave the way to your release from your diet prison.

Each day as I work with clients in my office, I hear new additions to the long list of reasons why people abuse food. As I offer you the most common ones, you may find many of them relevant. Perhaps you can add some reasons of your own. Don't be discouraged if you identify with *all* of them. It doesn't mean you are doomed to have a fat body forever — in fact, it is in your favor if you can be that honest with yourself. Remember you are re-educating yourself about the nature of weight loss and gain. You are learning to cultivate an entirely new way to relate to food. You are just a beginner at this point, so be kind and loving to yourself as you explore this material. You may have an extremely emotional reation to it.

In Chapter Six we will explore more fully how the subconscious mind operates. Meanwhile, you should know a few of the basics. The subconscious mind takes all instructions literally — it doesn't have the ability to make rational, intelligent decisions. Whatever your need, the subconscious mind will eventually find a way to meet it, even if it seems ridiculous to the intelligent, mature part of your conscious mind.

Now we're ready to look at the many reasons why people abuse food.

REASON 1: COMFORT

One of my teachers calls this the "Here Dear, Have A Cookie Syndrome." It starts when the sufferer is a little child. Something happens, like a minor fall, and she hurts her knee. Mother goes to her aid and says, "Here dear, have a cookie and it will feel better." Her young mind starts to associate food with comfort. Guess what she does, as an adult, when she and a loved one have a spat, or she flunks a history exam, or experiences any other upset which makes her cry out for comfort?

She eats! She eats for comfort.

REASON 2: WEIGHT IN THE WORLD

When we think of weight in the world, we usually think in terms of clout and personal power. Subconsciously, many people confuse physical weight and "weight" of influence on events and people.

For example, I once had a client who held a position on the Board of Directors of a large corporation. She felt conspicuous each time she entered the boardroom to attend a meeting because all her colleagues were men. She believed these men would not take her seriously if she showed up looking thin and feminine. She felt she had to maintain equal power by maintaining a stout, masculine body.

You don't have to be in a high-powered position like my client was for this reason to apply to you. It doesn't matter whether you are a homemaker, plumber, or farmer. It will be difficult to reduce as long as you equate extra weight with power or strength.

I find it interesting that quite a few people who attend my seminars first deny that the "Weight in the World" reason is part of their makeup. A couple of months down the road, however, many of them will say to me, "Remember reason number two? Well, I think I am using it."

Try to keep an open mind as you explore your reactions to this reason — and your reactions to the other reasons as well.

REASON 3: FOOD AS A SEX BARRIER

Many facets of sexuality are reflected through overeating. The incest victim, for example, may learn early on in life that if she gains a substantial amount of weight and makes her body unattractive, her molester will not be as interested. A person who fears sexual experiences for any reason will often gain weight in the thigh, hip, and pelvic areas, thus creating a prison to conceal and protect her genitals.

My client, Kathy, created her sexual prison to insure her marital fidelity. She had many sexual partners as a slim single woman and felt extremely guilty about it. Kathy was terrified she would be unable to maintain her monogamous vows when she got married. So she gained 30 pounds as quickly as possible and made herself less attractive to men, reducing the possiblity of an affair. It was only when she realized she had the ability to be faithful to one partner that Kathy was able to let go of her extra weight.

If you have experienced a painful sexual experience on a physical or emotional level, your subconscious may be saying "No more of this," and so you make yourself as unappealing as possible to the opposite sex. Ask yourself, "How safe do I feel sexually when I am at my perfect weight?" You may come up with some surprising insights.

REASON 4: HAVING SOMETHING YOUR OWN WAY

An overweight person will often have an extremely dominating person in her life who is constantly telling her what to do, how to spend her money, who to have or not have as friends, what time to be home, etc. She probably feels she doesn't have much say or independence in her life. A frequent response is to gain 25 pounds. It may be self-destructive, but it is something she can do over which no one else can possibly exert any control.

Everyone needs to have some independence in her life and will resort to extreme measures to achieve it. This is especially true for children with weight problems. Those extra pounds are screaming out, "You can't control my body! So there!"

REASON 5: TO BE OR NOT TO BE
LIKE SOMEONE ELSE

Most children find "heroes" they try to model themselves after. Imagine for a moment that it is dear Aunt Tilly whom you adore. She is witty, loving, generous, and makes the best chocolate chip cookies in the world. You had told yourself many times, "When I grow up, I am going to be just like Aunt Tilly." How wonderful if you had only inherited her wit and charm. Unfortunately, you have also been the beneficiary of her 250-pound figure because you instructed your subconscious mind to be *just like* Aunt Tillie.

This subconscious trap can also work conversely. Perhaps you and your mother were never able to agree on anything. You butted heads whenever you got the chance. More than likely, you vowed to be nothing like her; in fact, just as different as possible. But what if Mom has a slim, trim figure and you have been instructing yourself to *reject everything about Mom?* You probably don't get to have that great body.

You may have also been programmed by friends and family to emulate someone. Do you recall statements like, "Mary, if you don't stop eating that ice cream, you will look just like Uncle Fred." Good old Uncle Fred tips the scales at 280. So flip back through those pages in your memory book and see if you can recall any childhood vows and instructions.

REASON 6: REVENGE

My client, Rhonda, was 14 years old and lived in the Middle East where her father was a prominent diplomat. Her parents decided to send her to a boarding school in the United States. She was extremely angry about the "rejection" and felt compelled to exact revenge. Since her father placed great stock in personal appearance, Rhonda knew how she could "get" him. She became fat.

Think about your own situation. Who are you trying to "get" by being overweight?

REASON 7: THE SOCIAL BARRIER

Are you afraid to meet new people or to participate in social situations? Is it easier to just be the nondescript blob at a party? Or better yet, do you refuse the party invitations to stay home with the television and a Sara Lee cheesecake? If so, it looks as if you are using those extra pounds as a barrier to keep people from getting to know you. Your self-esteem is probably low and you are convinced no one would like you anyway. So why take the chance of being rejected and hurt? Sound familiar? If so, be sure to read and reread the upcoming chapter on improving your self-esteem. Accepting yourself unconditionally is the key to solving this problem. Everyone is intrinsically good, even if she tries to cover it up with a layer of fat.

REASON 8: INSULATION

I openly wept when my client, Cindie, told me of her childhood and her parents' constant, violent fights. The brawls were so terrifying that she would grab a loaf of bread, a bag of cookies, or anything else she could get her hands on and eat as rapidly as possible, unconsciously knowing the food would somehow block out the noise. She used this method of overeating to numb her battered body as well, for her mother didn't stop with violent words. She carried out her anger with physical abuse.

Cindie is not the only one who uses food to stop physical and emotional pain. A great amount of food does have a numbing quality. When a person eats more than the body can easily assimilate, the excess food sits in the stomach and ferments. This creates a sensation similar to drinking alcohol. You may experience drowsiness, numbness, and a general loss of energy which helps to insulate your feelings and keep the pain at bay.

REASON 9: THE ANGER STUFFER

Most of us were taught as children that anger is an inappropriate emotion. We were usually told, "Don't talk back to me! Just keep your mouth shut!" It probably comes from the same philosophical school as V.S. Bellamy's Victorian poem which admonishes that, "Children should be seen, not heard."

Anger is a healthy response to certain situations. Teaching your kids to repress anger is one of the greatest mistakes a parent can make. Suppressing anger means that it stays bottled up inside and can lead to all kinds of problems — such as overeating, for example. The overeater stuffs down her anger with food.

Virginia's experience is a good example of this. "I had just finished a very satisfying lunch and felt especially good about myself. The mail arrived and there was a letter from my father. I started to see red as I read his letter, for he was blaming me for something I didn't do. My mind nearly went blank with fury. The next thing I knew, I was in the kitchen frantically gorging on food I wasn't even tasting. I suddenly came to my senses and realized what I was doing: pushing down my anger with food. It was especially disgusting because I had just finished a good meal."

Virginia has now learned to express her anger in a positive way by being assertive and explaining her needs, eliminating the need to stuff it down with unnecessary food. Chapter Five provides some good techniques for dealing with anger in a positive way.

REASON 10: PARENTAL TEACHING

Many of our parents programmed our minds with beliefs which didn't always result in good eating habits. I think nearly every kid in America heard this one: "Clean up your plate, there are poor little children in India starving to death."

As an adult, this statement reverberates in your subconscious mind when you approach the end of a meal. You feel guilty that you are solely responsible for shoulder-ing the burden of some poor little kid's demise if you don't clean up that last bit of potatoes and gravy on your plate. The adult part of your mind, of course, is not conscious of that suggestion. But rest assured, it is there.

If you start paying attention to overweight people when they are eating a meal, you will notice that they clean their plate completely — often right down to the parsley garnish. Practice always leaving just a little something on your plate, assuring yourself it is OK.

Several women have told me that when their mothers explained the facts of life, they also threw in this little tidbit: "Dear, you are going to have to watch your weight when you start to have your period. Women always gain then." With that kind of instruction in your mind, you are going to expect an "inevitable" expansion and sub-consciously strive to meet that expectation.

If you come from a family that experienced a shortage of money, you may have heard the statement: "You had better get your fill of that tonight because it might be the last we have for a while." Or, if there were many family members sitting around the dinner table, you had to be fast to get your share. And if you wanted to save a little of your dessert to eat later, well, you knew there would be no chance of that. Someone would be sure to snitch it. These family situations create the need to "sneak" food, eat fast, and eat great quantities at one time.

As you can see by looking at old paintings, the fat look has often represented prosperity in our culture. This attitude still prevails to some degree. Take the case of the man who came from a family which didn't have enough to eat. He made a childhood vow (perhaps unconsciously) that when he had children, he would make sure they had *plenty* to eat. He certainly had good and loving intentions but he ended up with obese children. He would bring home sacks of goodies every night to prove his prosperity. Not wanting to disappoint Dad, the kids ate it all.

In some families, meal time was "bad news time." This was when the F in algebra was explained and you heard you couldn't go on the following weekend's campout. If this kind of negative conversation was the norm, you probably have negative associations with eating. When you re-experience these negative associations with food, you may have a tendency to go "unconscious" and lose all awareness of what you are eating. This makes you eat more and faster than is necessary simply because you don't want to be aware that you are eating at all.

Try to remember what your parents said about food, weight, your body, etc. It may be contributing to your weight problem. Please bear in mind, however, that it does not pay to blame your parents. Most of them had no idea of the impact these "harmless" little thoughts could have. And if you are a parent, please, please, re-read this section. Let's eliminate the need for your kids to suffer the woes of being overweight.

REASON 11: THE MOTHERLY IMAGE

Many women tell me they never had a weight problem until they had a baby. It is true, of course, that your body goes through a physical change, but it is not nearly to the extent that your *mind* changes. Just look at the difference in lifestyles between a parent and a non-parent. Your image of yourself may go from a sexy, spontaneous, carefree partner to a responsible, tied-down, weary mother.

What is the image we conjure up when we think of *Mom?* Not usually a slim, sexy, fashion-model type. Unconsciously we think of a soft, warm, ample lap to sit on and full, nurturing breasts. In other words, a plump, unassuming woman who is interested only in our welfare. These are the images impressed upon us as children, and they can still dominate unless we turn them around. Often a father will call his spouse "Mother," because she has also become "Mom" to him, or else he perceives her mother role is more important than her role as his wife. Being a good mommy, her image is wrapped up in the baby and she denies her own individuality. Her subconscious thought in this situation is that to be a good mother, she has to emulate that maternal image.

Not so, dear sisters! You can be a slim, attractive woman who has a life of her own — and still be a terrific mom.

REASON 12: LOOKING FOR SATISFACTION

"Are you satisfied with your life?" I asked Dorothy.

She lowered her chin and shook her head. Tears welled up in her eyes when she raised her face.

She is 49 years old — a vulnerable age for many women, when it is easy to succumb to a feeling of emptiness. Her children were in college, her husband was spending most of his time at work, and Dorothy was equally busy trying to find some satisfaction in her life by constantly eating. She was an intelligent, talented writer who had been unable to do get anything down on paper in a long time. She had lost the ability to do things for her own pleasure and satisfaction. She was always occupying herself with her kids' needs, her husband's needs, and her household duties. Dorothy needed to learn she had a right to satisfy herself with things other than food. She finally started to allow herself time to write short stories and to take classes at the local college. She learned to fill her void with positive things instead of with binging. And she started to lose weight, slowly and surely.

I mentioned that women of Dorothy's age are particularly susceptible to this problem — it is not restricted to her age group, however. Whether you are 18 or 80, if you feel dissatisfied with your life (or even a part of it), you may succumb to satisfying yourself with food.

REASON 13: GETTING SOMEONE'S ATTENTION

While counseling Amy, a 10-year-old girl, I began to see a picture of a very lonely and angry child. Her parents were busy professionals, always on the run to meetings, dinners, and appointments. Amy had a 14-year-old brother who was a whiz kid — good looking, popular, and a high achiever. She strongly sensed that her parents favored her brother. What little time and attention they could spare seemed to go to him. Being a kind and polite child, Amy tried to make all kinds of excuses for her parents' lack of attention. She often said things like: "It's important that Mommy takes her night classes so she will know more for her job," or "A lot of people need my daddy to help them, so I guess that is where he usually is."

Underneath all that sweetness was longing and rage, as well as a little mind ticking away in a plot to get her parents to notice her. She unconsciously chose a way that made her even more miserable: Amy got fat. In the process, she did manage to get attention. Her mother harped at her to go on a diet, her father voiced his disgust, and her brother called her "tubby."

Kids and adults need attention from the people they love. This need is so strong in humans they will go to any length to get it. Are you trying to get someone to notice you?

REASON 14: FOOD (LOTS OF IT)
KEEPS YOU HEALTHY

Do I ever remember this one from my childhood! If I mentioned a headache or a hangnail, my mother would have the chicken soup or the milk toast ready and shove a spoon in my hand. Her loving voice would be saying: "You probably just need a little something to eat." She came from the generation that believed "a fat baby is a healthy baby." Of course, we know differently now.

Many people still associate health, and even survival, with food or extra pounds. My client, Jean, was a classic example of this. Jean's mother became ill with diabetes when Jean was a teenager. The family relied on Jean to care for her mother during her illness. Jean watched her mother go from being slightly plump to being seriously underweight during her illness. When her mother died, Jean unconsciously connected weight loss with illness and ultimately, death. Jean used self-hypnosis during her weight-loss therapy. Each time she visualized herself slender, she became very upset and felt overwhelmed by the old fears of diabetes and death. This fear had been suppressed for years. After she worked with it for several months, she was able to associate slenderness with health and vitality. Only then was she able to lose her excess weight.

REASON 15: AVOIDANCE

Picture this: you are home and doing your best to ignore a pile of soiled laundry rivaling Mt. Everest. Every dish in the house is dirty and spilling all over the kitchen. And then there is that awesome tower of paperwork precariously balanced on the desk in your study. You want to tune out the whole mess, but there is a little voice deep inside saying, "You have to be productive and busy doing something or else you will become lazy." Laziness is something most people fear; they believe it is a sign of poor character.

There is a difference, however, between being lazy and having leisure time, but our naive subconscious mind can't make the distinction. So here you are, feeling the pressure to take care of all these chores. You also want to avoid them but are consumed with guilt because you feel lazy and don't really want to do anything at all.

What do you do? Your subconscious has the answer: *eat!* Eating satisfies all the needs in this situation. You get to avoid the tasks and yet "productively" engage yourself in something by eating. After all, eating is necessary for survival, right? Therefore you don't feel guilty about being lazy.

If you are using food in this way, you need to learn how to allow yourself free time. Practice just staring out the window if you feel like it. People need this "daydreaming" state to revitalize their creative juices. Let go of the stigma that you are worthless if you are not productive all the time. You might also re-evaluate how you organize your time. Schedule only what you can realistically manage in a day and let the rest go until tomorrow.

As you sort through all these reasons why people abuse food, keep in mind that most manifest themselves unconsciously — not through any rational means. This doesn't mean you can abdicate responsibility for your actions, and it doesn't mean your behavior is beyond your conscious control; it just means you don't have to feel like a fool for creating all these myths about food. In the following chapters you will learn ways to identify your reasons for overeating and how to resolve them.

REMINDERS FROM CHAPTER TWO

1. Excuses such as "I just love food," "I have a slow metabolism," or "I have overactive glands" are almost never the real reason for being overweight.

2. Food has a great psychological significance for most women.

3. It is imperative that you are honest with yourself when exploring the reasons you overeat.

4. Don't be discouraged if you identify with several reasons for overeating. Most people have more than one.

5. Be gentle and loving with yourself as you identify with the different reasons for overeating.

3

SELF-ESTEEM

Self-esteem is the most important quality a person needs to develop in order to achieve fulfillment and lead a sane, happy life. Overweight people usually have poor self-esteem. While most people can hide their insecurities and fears, the overweight person has no alternative: hers are on public display in the form of extra pounds. This "physical display of emotions" often means the overweight person is subjected to ridicule and humiliation by a lot of insensitive people.

OVERWEIGHT PEOPLE FACE DISCRIMINATION

The overweight person is made to feel like a second-class citizen. She is treated like a weak, inferior person

37

in all realms of her life. Even people who should know better seem to consider excess weight to be merely the result of exerting too little self-control.

You may have heard your doctor instruct you to just "push away from the table a little sooner and you will lose your extra weight." But you know you can't just push away from the table that easily, although you think the doctor should know what he is talking about. Fortunately, not all physicians are that insensitive.

And what about skinny Ms. Jones next door who is basically saying the same thing? In the face of such contempt, it is easy to view yourself as a cowardly slob with no will power. The doctor and Ms. Jones are not the only ones who are looking down their noses at you and your (God forbid) 35 extra pounds. Ignorance and an obsession with physical appearance has led our culture to unfairly persecute people with weight problems. No wonder overweight people suffer from poor self-esteem.

Since discrimination against overweight people is so prevalent in all realms of our society, it is the responsibility of *ALL* people (whether they are fat or thin) to overcome this prejudice and become more compassionate and understanding.

IT'S YOUR RESPONSIBILITY, TOO!

By slapping the offenders' hands, I don't mean to set up overweight people as victims. You can't allow yourself to wallow in self-pity because of others' insensitive attitudes. Only you can assume responsibility for building your own self-esteem.

There is often a big misunderstanding about what self-esteem is. Contrary to popular opinion, it is not conceit or egotism. Webster's dictionary defines self-esteem as "confidence and satisfaction in oneself." The key word here is *"in"*: *in* yourself, *in*side you. In other words, you like yourself, as you are.

The egotist, braggart, and blamer must get this approval externally. It must come first from others because she lacks this within herself. A person with good self-esteem doesn't have to tell the world how terrific she is. It is already apparent to everyone, especially her.

The origins of poor self-esteem usually can be found in one's youth. Children are often told that "it's not nice to brag about yourself." A child usually takes this as an indication that she is not a good enough person, thus breaking down any existing self-confidence.

OVEREATERS PUT THEMSELVES IN SECOND PLACE

It is not a selfish or unfair act to love yourself. If you don't care enough about yourself, why should anyone else? Receiving love from others always begins with being able to accept love from yourself. You deserve it.

Unfortunately, the overeater has tremendous difficulty loving herself. She will invariably put herself second, third, or tenth on her list of priorities. My client, Adel, is a good example. Adel takes great pride in being "Super Mom." She is a dedicated elementary school teacher, married to a professional man, mother of two children. She supports many community activities, and is a flawless homemaker. Adel is also angry, tired, and full of resentment. Why? Because she lets all these outside demands take priority over her own personal needs.

One situation she told me about typifies a normal day for her. As she prepared to leave school at the end of the day, her husband called to say he had an important meeting, and was unable to take their son to his music lesson as planned, and could she fill in? Adel also had an important appointment but dutifully put her needs aside and cancelled the meeting to chauffeur her son. After the music lesson, she arrived home, looking forward to relaxing with the evening paper. As soon as she walked in, her other son called.

"Dad must have forgotten to pick me up," he said frantically. "I am at little league practice. Please come and get me."

Once again, Adel denied her own needs, and picked up her son. When she returned home, her other son informed her that "Dad called and wants you to get ready to go to a business dinner with him." Adel cringed. All she wanted was some peace and quiet.

By this time, of course, she was not the least bit hungry, but the strain of conflict between her needs and her sense of obligation to so many others had made her eat...and eat...and eat. Since 4 p.m., she had been eating candy bars to soothe her frustration and potato chips to block out her anger.

Adel had put herself in second place and paid dearly for it. But she had also allowed the situation to develop. Her self-esteem was not strong enough to allow her to say "no." It was easy to blame her family but it was not their fault. She had to assume responsibility for making sure her needs were adequately met. Only she could do this.

Adel developed a strong sense of her self-worth over the months we worked together. She now realizes that it is not a selfish act to put herself first. In fact, she is now providing a much better role model for her children, and her husband has gained new respect for her. Best of all, she now likes herself. She now nourishes herself with her own love and respect — not with candy bars.

Adel repeatedly used two affirmations which can also help you: *"When I am a winner, others are, too"* and *"I can say 'no,' without risking loss of love."*

THINKING LOVING THOUGHTS

Take a moment and recall some of the negative things you have said about yourself. Think about how they have shaped your self-esteem. Are any of these statements yours?

"I am such a dummy."

"With my luck, I am sure to fail."

"I hate myself."

If you are programming your mind with lowly thoughts like these, that is right where your level of self-esteem will stay. You may not consciously realize you are saying these things, but with some time and some careful self-examinination, you can become aware of this kind of habitual thinking. By changing this kind of thinking, you can change your level of self-love. High self-esteem is the greatest gift you can give yourself. It is the foundation on which you can build a good life.

I have a list of fun exercises that can actually help increase your self-esteem. They are not in themselves a "sure cure," but they will assist you to become more aware of yourself and your needs (more on this in Chapter Eight). Before you read on, I want you to stop and close your eyes for a moment. Take a deep breath and say to yourself, *"I* (your name) *love myself."* You are now on the right path.

OTHER IMPEDIMENTS TO POSITIVE CHANGE

As you endeavor to lose weight and increase your self-esteem, there may be certain people who will unconsciously (or consciously) try to sabotage your efforts. My client, Lynn, saw this clearly as we did a visualization exercise in our support group.

I instructed the group to imagine themselves in a peaceful garden. They were to walk down a brick path until they came to a pond and then peer into the water until they could see the reflection of a person who may be trying to prevent them from losing weight.

Lynn saw her husband. He was holding a cake in his hands. She was amazed until she then began to recall other times she had lost weight. Her husband was constantly encouraging her to eat, in subtle ways, of course. He was feeling threatened by Lynn's emerging beauty and self-confidence. He was probably thinking subconsciously that if Lynn became too attractive, she would no longer want him, and it was far better to keep her overweight and dependent on him.

If you find someone in your life who is threatened by your physical and emotional change, let them know the relationship is safe. Be assertive and don't weaken your stance. You deserve this positive change you are creating in your life.

Children sometimes become somewhat frightened if their mother starts to lose weight. They often believe their mother is losing part of herself. Assure the children that you will always remain the good mother they appreciate and love.

Jealous mothers have often contributed to overfeeding their children. Reflect back on your childhood memories, and try to determine if your mother was ever jealous of you. Did she ever encourage you to eat food you weren't hungry for? Was she ever critical of your appearance, referring to you as plain, or pointing out flaws like a big nose?

Chances are she felt your father (her partner) may have lavished more attention and affection on you than on her. She could have been competing with you in some way. If she fed you enough, making you fat and unattractive, then she would regain some of that attention. This is usually an unconscious defense mechanism on the mother's part. While she may never have harbored any malicious intentions, her actions were still damaging.

If you conclude your mother was guilty of force-feeding you to insure her status within the family, then forgive and forget. It is only an unnecessary emotional burden for you now.

A FEW WORDS ABOUT CHOCOLATE...

Sweet, creamy, luscious chocolate. Ever thought about our love affair with chocolate? We love and hate it at the same time. Scientists have studied our passion for chocolate, and have come up with some interesting findings.

It seems that when a person eats chocolate, it triggers a chemical reaction in the brain similar to the feelings experienced when falling in love. That "all is well and warm in the world" feeling is certainly less intense when eating chocolate than when falling in love, but it is there in a subtler way. If you feel compelled to eat this particular sweet, you might want to ask yourself if you are using it as a substitute for love in your life.

These findings about chocolate's effect on human emotions further substantiates the theory that the majority of overweight women suffer from a lack of affection and love in their lives. They (and you) deserve real love, real affection. Accept no substitutes, not even chocolate!

NARROW ATTITUDES TOWARDS THIN PEOPLE

A good friend recently told me a story which illustrates prejudices overweight people frequently harbor toward thin people. My friend (who has a weight problem) works on the third floor of a tall building from which she and her co-workers watch the pedestrians on the street below. Whenever they see a thin woman walk by they make comments like, "With that body, she's got to be an airhead," and "She's beautiful, but oh so dumb." And they don't even know the the women they are putting down!

These women pay dearly for making such rationalizations. Subconsciously they are reassuring themselves into a trap. If they believe thin women are stupid, they will never be able to allow themselves to be thin because then they would have to become stupid, too. Don't let yourself succumb to this.

REMINDERS FROM CHAPTER THREE

1. Self-esteem is the most important element in creating a fulfilling life.

2. There is much discrimination against overweight people, which adds to low self-esteem.

3. Self-esteem is not egotism. It is not selfish to love oneself.

4. You must put yourself in first place.

5. Program your mind with thoughts of self-love.

4

WHAT ABOUT FOOD?

I remember standing in front of a supermarket bakery, making every possible effort to suppress the rage that was boiling up in me. I really wanted to devour a glazed twist but I also wanted to shrink my bulging thighs. It was the same old frustrating decision I faced dozens of times each day. And usually the glazed twist (or hot fudge sundae, hamburger, or french fries) won out in this contest of wills.

But something was different on this day. I was fed up with feeling powerless.

"I used to be thin," I told myself. "I deserve to be thin once more. I deserve to eat the foods I enjoy and still be thin!"

After this bold self-assertion, I marched right over to the counter and ordered one twist to go. To my utter amazement, I bought only one. With my head held high, I turned on my heel, marched to the car, and ate my beloved glazed twist.

I did more than just eat it, however. I enjoyed the taste, savoring every sticky morsel, feeling not a shred of guilt. I took my sweet time to finish it. This experience was the turning point in my compulsive eating career. This was the day I started to shed my extra pounds and my negative beliefs about food.

I ATE AND LOST WEIGHT!

As the months went by, I continued my practice of eating whatever I wanted. But the amount I wanted was different than before. I still enjoyed the same variety of foods, including the rich, high-calorie things that are always "no-no's" on a dieter's list. Now I couldn't finish one hot fudge sundae, let alone consume two or three as I could previously.

Miraculously, I was losing weight — maybe a pound or less a week, but I was losing it, and apparently for good.

SUCCESS — AT LAST!

I steadily lost weight during the year following my "enlightenment" — or at least my bold self-asserttion — at the supermarket bakery. I went through a surprising number of positive personal changes, increased my self-esteem, and rid myself of many negative attitudes.

I shrunk from a size sixteen to a size six in about one year. And my life started working better, in many ways. Many years have passed, and I have never gained back the weight. And I eat exactly what I want, when I want it.

My experience remained somewhat of a personal mystery until I went back to college and studied psychology. When I finally understood why I had been successful, I found other women who had also experienced the same thing. Then I knew my weight-loss method was no mere fluke — in fact, it seemed to be the only viable means for permanent weight loss. I have since worked to streamline the process and teach it to others.

BROWNIES ARE OK

Whenever I first talk to a client about food, I set up a little visual scene for her. I'd like you to try it.

Imagine you are at home, doing your usual chores. Suddenly, the craving hits: the image of a brownie pops into your mind. Moist, chewy, and chocolate. You can almost smell it. Your mouth waters.

"Are you kidding?" scoffs a little voice in the back of your mind. "Do you know what that will do to your hips?"

"You're right," you concede to the judgemental voice. "I'll just have some carrot sticks, instead."

So you eat the carrot sticks. A few minutes later, however, you still don't feel satisfied. That sultry image of the brownie comes back to haunt you. You fight it off with a virtuous thought about cottage cheese. You trot off to the refrigerator and eat some, but the yearning lingers. And so you continue to munch your way through the next couple of hours, eating half a sandwich, a piece of cheese, a peach. They're all good foods but they certainly don't hit the spot right now. The brownie still looms on the horizons of your mind.

And what have you done in the last three hours? You have consumed far more calories than are in one brownie. You feel bloated, disgusted, and discouraged. You have not accomplished anything positive by rejecting your natural craving for a brownie.

So how can you change this behavior to achieve a more positive result? You can play a little game with yourself to determine whether the particular food you crave is a "satisfaction food" or a "seducer food." When you get a craving for something, even a brownie, analyze the feeling. Is the brownie connected with any particular emotion? Anger? Loneliness?

If you can't detect anything other than just the simple need to eat the brownie, you can be pretty sure it will satisfy you totally. And you won't go on a binge.

THE SATISFACTION FOOD

So let's imagine another scenario. Go and get the brownie. Now sit down and examine its color and texture. Take a whiff and bask in the aroma. Eat it slowly and savor each delicious bite. Tell yourself, "It's all right for me to eat and enjoy this food." Don't allow yourself to succumb to feelings of guilt.

When you satisfy yourself with a brownie, you have eliminated all those superfluous calories in the other foods your body did not really want. You are now regaining some power over food, by deciding what you want and what you don't want. Your body knows which foods satisfy and will communicate this to you. I call these "satisfaction" foods.

So you can ask yourself: "Will this brownie (or whatever you crave) be satisfying?" If so, then eat it and enjoy it.

THE SEDUCER FOOD

There is another kind of food to be dealt with, however — the "seducer food." The seducer rears its ugly head in a scene like this: Once again you are home and going about your business. You say to yourself, "Gee, I feel hungry but I don't know what to eat." So you open the refrigerator and find some leftover chicken, some cherry pie, and a bit of fruit salad among the goodies.

You say to yourself, "Well, it all looks pretty good, so I'll just sample a little bit of everything." An hour later you are still looking for something to satisfy yourself but no particular food comes to mind. You have eaten and eaten, and you have been seduced. You've eaten food which has given you lots of calories, but no satisfaction.

The correct thing to do in this situation is to stop and examine your motives *before* you open the refrigerator. It may be that you don't really want food at all. If not, figure out what you really want. Dig into your head and be honest with yourself. Do you need comfort? Are you dissatisfied with your job or relationship? Try to determine what you need, and you will be able to exercise much more control over the situation.

Sometimes you will not be able to identify the need. It may be buried too deeply, or it may simply be too painful to deal with at the time. If that's the case, do something nice for yourself other than give into the seducer food. Take a bubble bath, call a friend, get a massage, write some affirmations (more on these later), go for a walk.

LIBERATED EATING

As you practice applying the satisfaction/seducer labels to various foods, you will discover a new feeling of power in your life. My clients often report a tremendous sense of relief when they begin to use this process.

When Wanda, a 54-year-old habitual dieter, heard about this process, she began to weep because she said it felt like an evil demon had left her body. Wanda initially found it difficult to apply this method to her eating habits because her lifelong programming said, "Rich, high calorie foods are fattening — even to look at!" But her determination was strong and she gradually exorcised this "demon." She eventually became quite adept at determining which foods she really should eat, regardless of their caloric content.

Understanding the differences between satisfaction foods and seducer foods allows you to eat what you really want. Eating what you want is the key to looking like you want. This is the behavior a naturally thin person uses to guide her eating, though it is usually carried out on a subconscious level. Eating according to the whims of your negative feelings (anger, fear, hurt) will not give you any long-term satisfaction.

NUTRITION HAS ITS PLACE

The examples in the previous paragraphs referred to such foods as brownies and sundaes — foods usually considered to be lacking in nutritional value. I often refer to these kinds of foods in a positive light because it is necessary to let go of the fear and negative associations we have built up towards them. They have too much power and influence on you when they are set in a class by themselves.

Of course, it is true you cannot live on cookies and candy alone and remain a healthy person. But if you have been deprived of these foods, you have probably built up a strong desire for them. So you must allow yourself to have what you want in order to get over the desire to have it all the time.

YOU HAVE THE RIGHT TO SAY NO!

Social situations often mean food. Picture this: you drop by to chat with a good friend. You aren't thinking about food at all; your mind and body felt totally satisfied. Your friend announces she has just made a raspberry cheesecake, and she proceeds to cut you a generous slice. She places it in front of you, awaiting your praise and gratitude.

Your mind runs through a barrage of thoughts. You don't want to eat it, but you don't want to offend your friend's sweet gesture. And the cheesecake looks incredibly delicious. You must be assertive with your friend and yourself. You don't have to hurt anyone's feelings to get your way in a situation like this.

"Oh, Jane, that looks fabulous but I am stuffed," you could say. "I had a big, late breakfast today. You are such a great cook that I don't want to miss this treat. Would you mind if I took it home? I want my taste buds to savor every beautiful morsel."

Everybody wins this way. Jane is completely flattered and you don't have to eat something you don't want. Best of all, you can eat the goodie later, when you really want it.

THE COOKIE CAPER

Terry, a young woman in my support group, told us how this method worked for her. She loved chocolate chip cookies. Being deeply submerged in the "diet consciousness" that plagues most of us, she cut them out of her life, except for binges (of course), and then each cookie was laced with guilt.

Terry bravely experimented with the theory that if you eat what you want, you will eat it in moderation. She allowed herself to eat some chocolate chip cookies — and each was consumed with less guilt than the one before. At the end of two weeks she found her craving for chocolate chip cookies had diminished considerably. Now she only occasionally wants a cookie or two and the binges have completely subsided.

She has also discovered that her body is starting to crave healthier foods: vegetables, fruits, and whole grains. Gravitating to wholesome foods usually happens when you stop resisting the "no-no's."

I have seen this work time after time. When you clear out negative thoughts about food and give your body a chance to speak for itself, it will direct you to good foods. This doesn't mean you won't want ice cream once in a while. You have to nourish the spirit as well as the body, and there are times when ice cream will do just that.

JUNK FOOD JEOPARDY

There has been a big swing towards good nutrition in the last decade, and rightly so. This seemingly positive interest, however, has backfired for some compulsive eaters. I have clients who tell me they feel so bad about eating something junky that they "make up for it" by eating more food, making sure it is the "right stuff."

It goes like this: Susan eats the jumbo bag of deep fried corn crunchies and washes it down with a large bottle of soda. The guilt! What would Adelle Davis say? Susan atones by fixing an avocado and sprout sandwich with homemade wheatberry bread. After the sandwich, she feels her body has some good ammunition to fight off that weak moment with the junk food.

Look at all the food Susan ate that she didn't really want or need. Her approach totally defeated its purpose. Here's a sensible alternative to Susan's remedy: simply stop after eating the junk food and rest assured your body will get the nutrition it needs — another time.

As you start to overcome your "diet-consciousness," it's important to learn more about good nutrition — not from a diet perspective but simply from wanting to know more about the vitamin content of whole grain vs. refined products, for example, or about cooking techniques that preserve rather than destroy nutrients.

Remember the old adage about moderation being the key to life? This is sound advice, and you can't go wrong when it is applied to food and nutrition.

TIME WILL TELL

As you gain more awareness about food, you will notice how your eating habits are greatly influenced by the time of day (or night) and the situation at hand.

Janet told me of her "problem time." Before her marriage, she would fix exactly what she wanted for dinner. If she felt like having peanut butter on toast, it was exactly what she ate. During this time she remained at her perfect weight and never had to worry about eating too much.

When she got married, she prepared large meals for her husband each evening. She felt duty-bound to sit down and eat with him. Janet started eating a great deal more than she ever had as a single person. She wasn't necessarily hungry for the evening meal, but it was a social time for her and her husband. Janet failed to understand that the quality of her social time could be preserved even if she ate her beloved peanut butter on toast while her husband enjoyed his steak and potatoes.

Family pressures are often self-imposed. If you find you are sacrificing your well-being in this way, discuss it with your family members and talk it out until you reach an amicable solution.

BOYCOTT EATING AT CAFE CRISIS!

Then there are the times you dine out at a place I call "Cafe Crisis." Think of all the mental speeches you give yourself before, during, and after a meal at a restaurant. You may experience acute anxiety, worrying about your level of self-control, and fear of the unknown.

Once seated in a restaurant, you check out to see if you know any of the other diners who might catch (fat) you *eating!* You scan the menu, questioning whether you should order the dieters' special (merely for appearances) or defy all good sense and plunge into the lasagna with garlic bread.

You glance around the room as you agonize over your decision, and it's just your luck that the snobby slim bean from the P.T.A. meetings is sitting at the next table.

You can't be caught with lasagna on your plate now. You can't risk having her see you commit such a heinous crime, so you raise your head proudly and order the "Skinny Salad Delight" (delight, my foot). You know that as soon as your feet hit the kitchen floor at home, you will be raiding the refrigerator for something *really* satisfying.

It's a cinch your evening out at the restaurant is totally unsatisfying. You feel a jarring blend of anger, embarrassment, deprivation, and failure. You round out this miserable state of mind with a solid dose of self-disgust after you have finished your post-restaurant binge.

You never have to put yourself through this unfair situation again. Eating is a national pastime, one of our greatest forms of pleasure and entertainment. Don't spoil the experience for yourself. Let's develop a positive attitude and a strategy for overcoming the "Cafe Crisis."

PLAN AHEAD

The first step is to consider the "satisfaction/seducer game" and determine which foods will satisfy you. Figure out what you are in the mood for, in terms of taste, texture, and variety. If you crave Mexican food, make reservations at a Mexican restaurant. Once you get there, examine the menu to determine what you really want — and don't worry about the thin women in the room. When you find something on the menu that hits the spot, order it. Tell yourself it is OK, you deserve it, and you have power over the cheese enchilada with extra salsa. It has no power over you.

Use the same technique as you did when you visualized the brownie. Examine the plate for the colors, textures, and combination of foods. If you discover something on the plate you didn't expect, move it away from the other food. Then cut the food up into three or four portions. This is easier if it is a sandwich but if it is something more complicated, like a bowl of spaghetti, just draw a line down the middle with your fork. Now eat one portion or side of the food. *Eat s-l-o-w-l-y!* Savor each bite so you can become more aware of the food's pleasurable aroma, flavor, and texture.

About halfway through the meal, stop, excuse yourself, and go to the restroom. Just take a few seconds, breathe deeply, and cast an admiring glance at yourself in the mirror. When you return to your meal, ask yourself how much more you really feel hungry for. There's a very good chance you won't need much more. When you determine that you are finished, call the waiter immediately and have him wrap the leftovers for you to take home. This kind of eating not only keeps you slim — but you will find that you can get two good meals for the price of one.

MONEY IS NO OBJECT

Don't be embarrassed to take food home from a restaurant. It prevents you from falling for the trap of thinking, "Restaurant food is expensive, so I should eat it all." *Never, never* use waste or economics as an excuse to eat food you are not hungry for.

Use these restaurant habits at home and you will find that meals become truly enjoyable experiences. You become part of the cafe society instead of a cafe casualty.

THREE DAILY MEALS DON'T SQUARE

In elementary school, our nutritional training (such as it was) advised eating three hearty meals each day: breakfast, lunch, and dinner. That routine may be fine for some (such as Olympic athletes and heavy construction workers), but certainly not all. I oppose any standardized routine that regiments people, regardless of individual needs. What if you are not hungry for dinner at 6 p.m.? What if you prefer combining breakfast and lunch at 11 a.m.?

Habits like this are usually frowned upon as irregular and unhealthy. Yet the human body has an innate wisdom when it comes to determining its needs. Your body will tell you when it needs nourishment and when it's time to eat. You have to experiment and learn to listen to your body. Then you can figure out your own meal routine, which will probably vary from time to time.

My own routine lately, for instance, has been to have just tea or coffee until about 10:30 a.m., and then a light meal or series of small snacks. I eat something pretty hefty around 1:30 p.m., usually some protein and starch. I eat a light dinner of whatever I want about 6:30 p.m. This is no controlled eating plan that I consciously devised. It came from listening to my own body's signals and my individual needs. I imagine it will change somewhat in time — to what I don't know. I'll just have to wait until I get the next message.

WORKING AROUND THE 9-TO-5 ROUTINE

You may find your work schedule creating a conflict with the way you would like to eat. By using your ingenuity, you can always figure out some way that you can win.

Many working women experience the kind of situation that a client of mine named Ruth complained about. She told me that she was forced to eat breakfast at 7 a.m. or go without in order to arrive at her job on time. She usually opted to go without since she could not easily face eating at that early hour. But then she became quite hungry about 9:30 a.m. and the only available food was candy from vending machines or the occasional donuts someone brought in. Ruth felt stuck. She didn't like eating candy or donuts because they made her feel hyperactive; but she also knew if she didn't eat something, she would be so ravenous by lunch time that she would eat twice as much as she needed.

By the time Ruth came to me, she had created such frustration around her work and eating schedule that she was ready to quit her job. She had steadily gained weight simply because she was no longer listening to her body's signals.

Together, we found a very simple solution. I suggested that Ruth carry raisins and almonds to work and eat some whenever she felt hungry. This combination satisfies the sweet tooth and also provides something solid to "stick to the ribs." Both raisins and almonds are nutritious, and a small amount alleviates hunger. They are also small enough to eat discreetly. Ruth has now varied her morning snack with other dried fruits and nuts.

It didn't take much to get Ruth back into good eating habits. Had she attempted to find the answer to her problem as soon as she recognized it, she could have spared herself the weight gain and the frustration.

If you find your work schedule creating a conflict with your meal patterns, use your ingenuity to figure out a satisfying solution to the problem.

KIDS ARE GREAT TEACHERS

As you gain more knowledge about good eating habits, be sure to apply it when you are teaching your kids how to eat. In fact, it is often better for you to let your kids teach you how to eat than for you to attempt to control their natural eating patterns. What if your child wants a peanut butter sandwich at 4:30 p.m.? You probably refuse because it will spoil her appetite for dinner. What is wrong with letting your child eat what she wants at 4:30 p.m. and then eat very little, maybe even nothing, at the regular dinner time?

I think we adults all too often mess up our kids' innate wisdom about eating. Certainly good, nutritious food should be emphasized, but try to relax and see what you can learn from the smart little kid sitting next to you at dinner.

ANXIETY AFTER WORK?

Many women say another problem time they face during the day is the first minute they get home from work, often feeling tired, rushed, anxious, or tense.

The normal routine is to immediately grab something — anything — to eat and then, without stopping to catch your breath, to launch into preparing the evening meal. As you slice the cheese for the casserole, a little song is playing in your head that entirely bypasses your conscious, adult mind:

"Two for the dish, one for me; a handful for the pot, a pinch for me; a cup for the bowl, a lick for me." On and on it goes, until you have consumed enough for a full meal by just munching your way through the preparation.

This wouldn't be so bad if you stopped there, but you eventually find yourself eating another meal at the dinner table. How can you stop this undesirable routine?

First, you have to become more aware of your mental state when you come home from work. Are you frazzled after the long day? Are you angry or frustrated about something at work? Go immediately to your bedroom or some private place and remove your work clothes. Slip on a bathrobe and lie down on the bed or sit in a comfortable chair. Close your eyes for just 10 minutes, or longer if you can manage it. Take a few deep breaths and think good thoughts. Instruct your family or room-mates that this is your special time and you are not to be disturbed.

After relaxing, change into some comfortable clothes, and *then* start your food preparations. This simple exercise will calm you down so you can be conscious of what you are doing and able to resist constant snacking while fixing the meal.

One woman realized that she entered her house through the kitchen each time she came home from work. The presence of food seemed to trigger a reaction to eat. She decided to start entering her house through the front door, which led into her living room, thereby avoiding the subliminal suggestion to eat.

NIGHTTIME MUNCHIES

All you late night eaters are a special group with a common denominator: most of you are unable to cope with relaxation, lazy time or solitude.

Picture this: everyone in your household is in bed, set-tled in with a book, or watching television. You find yourself cruising back to the kitchen in search of some-thing to eat. As you finish fixing a bowl of Cheerios with milk and sugar, you decide to do one of two things: go public or stay in hiding.

If you are feeling especially brave this evening, you join your partner, who is watching television. You feel ready to deal with snide comments like, "What are you doing eating? — we just finished dinner!" or, "Oh well, you can stuff down your anger with a second bowl of Cheerios."

Most of your eating is done in the closet, however, meaning you sneak the food so no one will see you. What you are really demonstrating is that you feel guilty when you are relaxing; you need to feel productive, and eating is an activity that protects you from seeing yourself as a lazy person. Eating gives you much-needed time with yourself to just relax and think of nothing important.

It is imperative for you to have time to yourself — time to just sit back and do nothing. But you don't have to justify that time by eating. Try risking an evening without your late night snack. Acknowledge to yourself that you deserve this lazy time, and you are still a good, productive, and caring person... even if you just sit and gaze at the stars for an hour or more.

MAKING EATING A BEAUTIFUL EXPERIENCE

As former dieters, most of you have developed a love/hate relationship with the physical process of eating. To help overcome any negative associations, try to make it as aesthetically pleasing as possible. Make a big deal out of eating something when you are hungry. Get out your best china, crystal, linens, and silver. Put some flowers on the table before you sit down.

Enjoy the process of eating, and pamper yourself with the beauty surrounding you. You are worth the trouble. Eating food should be a joyous experience. The more you acknowledge this, the less guilt and fear you will have — and by now you know that guilt and fear lead to eating much more than is necessary. Do this exercise regularly and enjoy it!

REMINDERS FROM CHAPTER FOUR

1. When you are about to eat, ask yourself whether it is a seducer food or a satisfaction food.

2. As you come closer to eating like a naturally thin eater, learn more about good nutrition.

3. Don't try to "cancel out" the junk food you just ate by eating good food that you really don't want.

4. Analyze your "problem time," and use your creative imagination to find a solution.

5. Make sure you have some time to relax by yourself.

5

YOUR PERFECT WEIGHT

When women lose weight, their minds frequently tend to lag behind their bodies. So many times a client will complain to me about her "fat" body when all I can see is a perfectly fine figure standing before me. It is obvious that her self-image is distorted. She really does see extra pounds whenever she looks at herself in a mirror. This image problem is typical of a woman who indeed has been overweight and then reduced through diets, diet pills, fasting, or other unnatural methods.

Her method of weight loss did not include a mental change, only a physical one. Let's say that her top weight was 175 and her perfect weight is 130. At 175, she frequently looked in the mirror and said, "I hate weighing this much." She would then go to the closet and pull out clothes that fit a 175-pound figure. She also got on the scales (maybe several times a day) and each time had to face that dreaded number 175! With this reinforcement, she easily programmed her mind into believing she was a 175-pound woman.

Then she went on a papaya and pineapple diet. Though she managed to lose the extra 45 pounds she didn't need, the magic fruits she consumed didn't do a thing for the "fat" picture in her mind. Her 175-pound body had become so familiar that her subconscious mind expected her to remain that way, no matter which diet she went on. As a result, she allowed her weight to slowly creep back up, thus fulfilling her own expectations.

"I wouldn't do that to myself!" you are probably thinking. But you probably would... and there's a good chance you have already done it several times. Remember, this is a battle that takes place on a subconscious level: you are not conscious of what you are doing. On the conscious level, it just seems like you have been indulging in too many goodies.

YOUR PERFECT WEIGHT

You can avoid this common trap. The first step is to *determine the correct weight to mentally associate with your desired self-image.* Choosing the goal weight is confusing for many women because it is entirely an individual matter. The most important thing to remember, however, is to set your mental sights on the perfect weight right away. Don't set intermediate goals. My client Nancy and I learned this the hard way.

Nancy weighed 170 pounds when she came to see me. She felt she would like to weigh 125. She was a model student and consistently worked with the techniques I taught her. We both agreed that setting intermediate weight goals might prove easier. Nancy set about programming her mind to believe that she was a 145-pound woman. She easily reached that goal, but then she suddenly stopped losing weight. After several frustrating weeks, she finally got over the hump and continued to lose until she attained her perfect weight.

After analyzing her situation, we realized that Nancy's mind had so firmly believed that she would be 145 pounds that it was not about to let go of the interim goal until she could firmly implant a new one. Her experience cost her a great deal in time, anxiety, and confidence. Fortunately, her determination won out, and she overcame the problem.

YOU ARE ONE OF A KIND

You may think that you will find a chart prescribing your perfect weight on the next page. Not in this book! Setting your perfect weight in your mind is a highly personal decision, and there are many individual considerations to keep in mind. Have you ever seen a weight chart that takes your particular lifestyle and emotional needs into consideration?

My client Candace is a perfect example. She weighed 183 pounds when she first consulted with me, but she always thought she should tip the scales at no more than 127. After all, the insurance company's chart said so. She got her weight down to 145. She felt wonderful, looked terrific, and loved the way she could now wear clothes. Her subconscious mind, however, kept up the pressure. She had to weigh 127 pounds.

We analyzed her lifestyle. She loves to wear loose, flowing clothes. She hates vigorous activities. She is married to a man who adores her and her body. Candace is an extremely feminine woman who knows how to wear makeup and fix her hair. She is also in perfect health. It finally dawned on us that her perfect weight is 145.

I also know women who prefer to be somewhat under the "normal" weight for their height. *The most important thing is that you are healthy and happy with your weight.*

Consider the things that Candace did. Are you athletic, or do you prefer a romantic walk on the beach for your exercise? What kind of clothes do you like to wear? Do you have any specific health problems? How do *you* feel about your body?

THE CHOICE IS YOURS ... AND YOURS ALONE

As you start to get in touch with the body image that is most satisfactory for you, you will probably become more aware of many of the outside pressures which influence you and separate you from what you really want.

The Duchess of Windsor once said, "No woman can be too rich or too thin" — and everyone has ever since taken this glib remark far too seriously. The media, for example, inundates us with suggestions that we must be thin! thin! thin! to be happy, successful, and attractive. They use the female body to sell everything from tires to diet soda. Unfortunately, these ads also sell us on the idea that our bodies are the key to power. There are two prerequisites for holding this key to power: our bodies must be beautiful and they must be thin. No wonder we women are so often obsessed with being thin.

We also get conflicting messages from women's magazines. On one page we see an article about dieting, clearly conveying the message that "if we are thin, men will love us." The facing page invariably features a spread on "Fabulous Chocolate Desserts," subtly conveying the message that when we provide lots of wonderful food for our families, they love us much more.

Confused?

All this media programming will continue until women themselves say *NO!* We cannot place all the blame on Madison Avenue advertising, even though they so powerfully reinforce so many of our cultural values. It is up to us to reject this externally imposed pressure. It is only by assuming responsibility for what we as individuals want our bodies to become that we can disengage ourselves from this obsession with being thin.

USING IMAGINATION TO ATTAIN YOUR IDEALS

After you have thoroughly explored your goals and targeted your perfect weight, you need to know how to prepare your mind to accept it. My clients have been very creative with their methods. One woman purchased a beautiful gold necklace with a pendant that said "124." It was a constant reminder each time she looked at herself wearing it. Others have printed up a business-size card with the affirmation, "I, (use your name), now weigh (your perfect weight) pounds." They carry the card around with them everywhere. If they are waiting in the dentist's office, for example, they pull out the card and look at it for a few seconds. Some keep the card in their purses so they will be reminded of their ideal weight whenever they open their bags. A few clients tape the card to their mirrors or refrigerators or other prominent places in their homes. Another effective trick is to remodel your scale — if you haven't thrown it out already. Write your perfect weight and tape it across the register so that each time you weigh in you will see your dream number smiling back at you. That feels just great!

MAKING A TREASURE MAP

Another fun and favorite method I recommend is called the treasure map. It is essentially a visual affirmation which sends the message to your subconscius mind that the picture before you is the way you are really supposed to look.

All you need is a piece of construction paper, some old magazines, a pair of scissors, paste, pen, and imagination. Keeping your own individuality in mind, cut out pictures of a body that resembles your ideal. If you are the sporty type, for example, choose an athletic body with a tennis racquet in her hand instead of a woman dressed in pearls and lace. Don't settle for something that is not you.

When you have made the choice, paste the picture on construction paper. Use an old photograph of your head to paste on top of the body. Then cut out favorite words or sentences pertaining to your relationship to your body and to food: "Losing weight is easy," for example, or "I feel terrific!" You can also put your favorite affirmations and perfect weight goal on the treasure map.

One woman I know only wanted to change her waistline and tighten her too-large tummy. She decided to cut out pictures of "good" tummies and put them on her map.

Put the treasure map some place where you will see it often so it will become implanted in your subconscius mind. Put it in a private place if there are people in your household who might think you are on the verge of "slipping off the deep end." You don't need any skeptics to undermine your efforts.

THINKING THIN!

The simple act of visualization is a very effective tool for changing your mental and physical image. Take just 10 minutes each day to lie down, breathe deeply, and allow your mind to float down that stream of consciousness (more on this in Chapter Eight). Envision yourself at your perfect weight, notice the clothes you have on, and observe your surroundings, making them as lavish and beautiful as you want. Now see yourself at your perfect weight in your real life, going to your job, seeing friends, meeting new people. This process will enable your subconscious to get used to the new you. When you do attain your weight goal, your subconscious will feel safe and comfortable with it.

A SIZZLING LOVE AFFAIR WITH YOUR BODY

Now it's time to start loving the body you see whenever you peer into the mirror. Quit persecuting yourself each time you see your reflection. Remember, if you continue to say, "Ugh, look at those bulging thighs," your mind will take that as an instruction to hold onto the bulges. If you say, "I hate my body," you are only putting yourself down. The end result is a diminished self-esteem which reinforces your subconscious mind to believe you are an unworthy person who doesn't deserve anything good, especially being slender.

Here is an example of how you can use the mirror for positive results. Several years ago, I still had my "saddle bags" on my thighs after losing my excess weight. They were certainly not as large, but still too much for my taste. I was still not comfortable in a bathing suit. I decided to do something about it, so I started looking in the mirror each day when I got dressed. I pulled the excess flab to the back as much as possible, saying to myself, "Karen, your legs are really beautiful. They are smooth and slender. You look great in your bathing suit."

At first, I was far too conscious of feeding myself a big line. As the weeks progressed, however, I started to believe myself more and more. When summer did arrive, I put on my bathing suit and realized that my legs *actually were* looking as good as I had been suggesting.

Close friends who were unaware of my mirror suggestions even commented on how nice my legs looked. My subconscious had been successfully programmed to believe in "nice legs for Karen," so my body was able to go ahead and change as per my instructions.

Give your body a break, love it and it will return the good deed. Most of all, remember it is *your* body. It does not belong to your family, the media, your employer, your partner, any group or institution. Make it the way which best suits *you*.

REMINDERS FROM CHAPTER FIVE

1. Program your mind to believe you are your perfect weight *now*.

2. Select a goal weight that is right for you and your lifestyle, not what is shown on a chart.

3. Do not set intermediate goal weights.

4. Resist outside pressure from the media. Take full personal responsibility for what *you* need in your body size.

5. Love your body in your mirror and in your mind.

6

HOW YOUR MIND WORKS

"Everything I eat turns to fat."

I often hear fragments of guilt-ridden diet conversation like this coming from nearby tables when dining out in restaurants. I can hardly keep myself from jumping up from the table.

"Stop!" I want to shout, "Don't you know what you are doing to your body with that negative statement?"

But I contain myself, of course, and silently pray the person will soon discover the creative power of her mind.

Few people really understand the power of the mind. The newly emerging, powerful belief that *you create your own reality* should not be scoffed at or underestimated in any way. Ironically, I was overcome with self-disgust when I first realized the validity of this statement.

"If I create my own reality," I asked myself, "then why did I make myself fat and miserable?"

Suddenly, something occurred to me which changed my life: if I could make myself fat, then I also must have the power to make myself slim! And I could be rich instead of poor, and loved and not rejected. The trick was to learn how to use my mind's power for, not against, myself!

THE CONSCIOUS AND SUBCONSCIOUS MIND

In order to make your mind work in positive ways, you must first understand that you are dealing basically with two very different components of your mind: the subconscious and the conscious.

The conscious part of your mind can be described as rational, intelligent, and "adult-like." It is through the conscious part of your mind that you are aware of your thoughts and actions. The conscious mind has the capacity to make mature decisions and value judgements by evaluating the available information which pertains to any given situation.

By contrast, the subconscious mind operates on a reactive level. It does not have the ability to make judgements, and it takes everything literally. The great psychoanalyst and philosopher, Carl Jung, referred to the subconscious as "child-like." Think of your subconscious as a five-year-old kid inside your head who is attempting to run your life according to her own values and perceptions.

You can also compare the subconscious to a computer. Like a computer, the subconscious receives programming without any attempt to rationalize or analyze it on an intellectual level. A computer will easily accept the premise that $2 + 2 = 5$ if you program it that way. Your subconscious will believe you if you tell yourself, "It's impossible for me to lose weight unless I starve myself."

Remember the statement, "Everything I eat turns to fat"? Just imagine what your subconscious mind is doing with that one! Like a child, the subconscious thrives on familiarity and repetition. The more you repeat a statement — any statement — the deeper it is implanted in your subconscious mind, and the more quickly it manifests itself in your life. Subconscious programming is a self-fulfilling prophecy.

Now is the time to start feeding your conscious mind with positive thoughts so your subconscious mind will take *those* literally, thereby providing some positive results. As you become aware of your "instructions" to yourself, you will be amazed to discover how these thoughts have been affecting your life.

YOU ARE WHAT YOU THINK

Creating one's own reality through thought is not exactly a new fad. In the Bible's *Epistle to the Romans*,

12:2, the Apostle Paul advised, "Be ye transformed by the renewing of your mind." This belief is not restricted to Christianity, for the Buddhist Holy Book, *Dhammapada (The Path of Teaching),* agreed, "We are what we think, having become what we have thought."

Once you begin to digest this concept, you will realize the key to using it for your own welfare. *You* are this key. You are the most powerful instrument for your own change.

Don't despair if you are feeling disgusted with yourself. I felt this, too. If you had the power to get yourself to where you are now, then you also have the power to place yourself somewhere else.

Imagine that your life up to this point has been memorialized in the pages of a book. You read it, thinking it will never be a best-seller. The main character (you) is overweight, doesn't like herself, and her life is dull, dull, dull.

Equipped with the understanding that you create your own reality with your mind, you can write a sequel to the first book. You can make your main character slender, healthy, happy, exciting, and anything else you desire, because you have the power to guide yourself into any direction you want. *You* are the author of your own story, the programmer of your own computer. *You* are the parent of your inner child and ultimately responsible for your thoughts. In other words, you can direct your life and free yourself from obsessive behavior toward food or anything else.

I get so excited when I talk to groups about the power of the mind! It is thrilling to see them begin to use this information and really change their lives. When they start to understand their potential for change, their enthusiasm generates enough electricity to light up New York City!

AFFIRMATIONS: THE KEY TO YOUR MIND

You are probably wondering how to initiate this change. There is a very simple process which I have found to be an exceptionally powerful mental tool: *Affirmations*. An affirmation is *a positive sentence which you put into your subconscious to get a positive result.*

Notice that I describe this process as simple. Many people conclude that a simple process is ineffective because they have been led to believe one must struggle and work very hard to get good results. This is not always so.

Bear in mind that we are trying to appeal to a five-year-old residing in the subconscious mind. This kid won't respond to difficult or complicated instructions, but she will easily digest a straightforward affirmative sentence. Go back to the thought, "Everything I eat turns to fat." Since you do not want to achieve the results of this statement, you should change it to something like this: "Everything I eat turns to health and vitality."

HOW TO USE AFFIRMATIONS

1. Say them in your mind. We say affirmations in our minds all the time; they are the inner dialogue we carry on with ourselves. Now is the time to become more aware of your mental chatter and place positive statements in the mental script. Become aware of your inner thoughts — whenever you catch yourself indulging in a negative thought, consciously stop it and replace it with a positive one.

2. Say them in a mirror. Try to really see yourself the next time you gaze into a mirror. Notice your eyes, your facial expression, and your entire face. Say a positive affirmation while looking straight into your eyes. You may discover that you try to avoid eye contact with your own image. Stay with it and you will soon begin to feel more comfortable with yourself. Start the day by saying, "I love you," while looking at yourself in the mirror.

3. Say them with a friend. If you have a supportive and understanding friend, ask her to do some affirmations with you. Simply maintain eye contact and take turns repeating an affirmation to one another. My husband, daughter, and I frequently help each other with affirmations. If my daughter is anxious about a test at school, for example, our affirmation session will go along the following lines:

"Heather, math tests are easy for you," I will say. "You always have the right answers."

"Yes, math tests are easy for me," Heather will answer. "I always have the right answers."

Exchanging affirmations with another person is also a great way to pass the time while driving for long periods of time. (I don't recommend sustaining prolonged eye contact with the driver, however.)

4. Record them on tape. Listening to affirmations on tape is especially convenient if you are short of time. Use your affirmation tapes in the car, while doing housework, or while doing any other mundane activities which require little concentration. It is also helpful to simply lie down and relax while listening to them. You can record your own or purchase professionally made affirmation tapes. (Mine are offered at the back of this book.)

5. Write them. The human mind learns 70 percent more efficiently by working with the writing process. Buy a notebook to use exclusively for affirmations. For seven days, write three affirmations at least ten times each. Then drop that set and choose another three for the next week. You may want to do more than three per day but try not to do too much; you could easily overwhelm yourself into stopping them altogether.

Save all of your written affirmation notebooks. It is fun and encouraging to go back to them and see how your efforts have paid off.

You will probably find that you utilize all these affirmation methods sooner or later, and perhaps even invent some of your own. Whatever your choice, make sure you practice them on a consistent basis. It's virtually impossible to learn anything with a hit-and-miss approach.

AFFIRMATIONS WORK!

While discussing affirmations in one of my classes, a 75-year-old woman's eyes lit up.

"So that was what my mother was doing all those years," she said. "I remember her standing in front of her mirror every day saying, 'I weigh 140 pounds.' Sure enough, she always did."

Another woman reported exciting results with one particular affirmation. She called me 10 months after attending one of my workshops.

"Karen," she said, "The only thing I have done as a result of your workshop is to use the affirmation, 'I like myself unconditionally.' I have said it each day and lost 25 pounds!"

She did not consciously try to cut down on her eating, but the power behind her affirmation had created some subtle changes which she had not detected.

BELIEVE IN AFFIRMATIONS AND YOURSELF

Sometimes affirmations work suddenly and dramatically; others are slow and subtle. Have faith, for affirmations do work. The subconscious may try to reject anything new, even though your new "program" is more positive. Familiar beliefs, albeit destructive, are "safe and comfortable." This is where faith comes in. Don't let yourself become discouraged. You invented those negative beliefs and you can also destroy them.

SAVE ON YOUR PSYCHIATRIC BILLS — ANALYZE YOURSELF

Affirmations are also a powerful tool for self-analysis. Carol, a beautiful German woman, told me of her insights while she practiced affirmations. She was 100 pounds overweight and couldn't figure out why, though one problem area in her life was readily apparent: she felt uncomfortable around others in professional and social situations. The nature of her job, however, forced her to constantly interact with other people.

Carol wrote the affirmation, "I now feel comfortable when I am with other people," but she detected a resistance in the inner recesses of her mind which said, "Oh, no! I will never feel safe around men!" She was perplexed by her reaction, as she had always believed her aversion was to people in general — not men in particular. The negative reaction to her affirmation gradually became clearer until she understood the reason. For the first time in years, she was able to recall an unpleasant scene from her childhood.

Carol remembered opening the bathroom door to find her father standing in his underwear. Carol was severely beaten for "peeking." Her father brutally taught her that sex was a "dirty, sinful" act.

This painful recollection enabled Carol to understand that she had been shielding herself from men with her extra 100 pounds. This was her way of avoiding the "dirty, sinful" sex trap.

She created new affirmations:

"I no longer need extra weight to protect myself from men because men and sex are safe."

"I am now comfortable and safe with my own sexuality."

When Carol finally banished her negative thoughts about sex, she found she no longer needed her extra 100 pounds for protection. Like Carol, it is important for you to be aware of your reactions to affirmations and then use them to get to the bottom of your weight problem. The following example illustrates how this can be done:

Affirmation: "I enjoy being slender and attractive."

Reaction: "Oh, no! Men always watch me, even stare. This scares me."

After analyzing your reaction to this affirmation, a new one could be created which would be more helpful:

"Being slender and attractive is safe for me," or "I expect and receive respect from men, even when I am slender and attractive."

CREATING QUALITY AFFIRMATIONS

As you create new affirmations for yourself, keep a few simple rules in mind:

1. Keep your affirmations in the present tense. If you say, "I will lose weight," instead of "I *am now* losing weight," your mind will literally interpret it as something to do in the future.

2. Keep the affirmations positive. Tell yourself "I am now well," instead of "I am no longer sick," thereby eliminating any negative connotations.

3. Give yourself any due credit when your affirmations come true. People will frequently say, "Oh, well, it would have happened without the affirmation." This may be true, but the the more you believe in the power of your affirmations, the more effectively they will work for you.

As you become more familiar with the affirmation process, start creating your own. If you get stuck on the correct wording, remember to take the negative thought you want to get rid of and make it positive. For example:

Negative thought: "Losing weight is difficult for me."

Affirmation: "Losing weight is easy for me."

Here are some sample affirmations to help you get started:

Weight and body image:

1. I enjoy being slim and attractive.

2. I now expect to lose weight and keep it off.

3. I deserve to be slender and healthy.

4. I have the right to be thin.

5. I am now willing to succeed at being thin.

6. I am so successful now, I no longer need to get even by being overweight.

7. My body size has nothing to do with my effectiveness in the world, therefore it is safe to be slim.

8. I am capable and respected, even if I am thin.

9. Everything I eat turns to health and vitality.

10. I feel good whether or not I eat.

11. I now have successful relationships whether or not I am thin.

12. The more I love my body, the more beautiful it becomes.

Self-esteem:

1. I love myself unconditionally.

2. I feel good about being me.

3. I am gentle and loving with myself.

4. I am whole, I am complete, and I am perfect just as I am now.

5. I now receive assistance and cooperation from other people.

6. I am safe, supported, and loved.

7. I expect approval and acceptance because I like myself.

8. The more I like myself, the easier it is for others to like me.

9. I have the right to say no without losing anyone's respect.

10. I now attract loving, accepting people.

11. I enjoy my own company.

12. I now feel peace of mind.

Perhaps the most important affirmation of all is this one: *My affirmations work!*

REMINDERS FROM CHAPTER SIX

1. Through your thoughts, you create your own reality.

2. Your subconscious mind is like a computer; it takes everything you say or do literally.

3. Taking full responsibility for your thoughts allows you to direct your life more effectively.

4. Affirmations are a powerful tool in creating positive results for you.

5. Affirmations can be used for self-analysis.

7

THE JOY OF EXERCISING

I know what you are thinking:

"Here it comes again — another sermon about the joys of exercise from a fanatic born-again athlete."

I used to feel the same way. And the guilt was far worse than not exercising.

I tried two exercise plans for each of my dietary misadventures. I faithfully followed Jack LaLanne (for two days) on television. Then I tried a stationary exercise bike, which was just as discouraging, though it lasted two days longer than Jack LaLanne — mainly because I felt guilty about the money I spent on it. I have tried jumping rope, dancing in my living room, aerobic dancing classes, weight lifting, and a myriad of other failures.

None were right for me. This is the key element to finding a suitable exercise program: it must suit *you!* It must also be fun. I know of other women who have tried some of these exercises and *they* have succeeded — only because they were enjoyable and suitable for them.

DESIGNING YOUR OWN EXERCISE PROGRAM

Ask yourself what you want to get out of your exercise program, as well as what might best fit your personality, needs, and skills. Analyzing the excuses you make is sometimes a good way to choose the best kind of exercise for yourself. I have heard women say they hate to go outside of their homes because they feel embarassed wearing shorts, or they have small children at home who can't be left alone.

The solution in this case might be a mini-trampoline: it's fun, and you can use it in your home and watch television or listen to your stereo while exercising. Mini-trampolines are also easy on your joints, which is why many doctors recommend this device for elderly people.

If you feel overwhelmed by extreme physical exertion, long walks may be your style. They often can develop into alternate periods of running and walking, which can prove to be very satisfying for some people. Please remember you don't have to run a marathon the first day to be successful. A walk at a steady, rhymthic pace is very good for your body and soul.

You may be justifying your inertia with excuses about health problems or physical handicaps. My medical consultants say there is usually no impediment to engaging in some form of exercise which will not aggravate your handicap. You can find the appropriate form of exercise with your doctor or physical therapist's guidance.

You don't have to be athletic, young, or strong to exercise successfully. Just use your imagination and find the right way for you. One of my most successful clients was a woman confined to a wheelchair.

If you have little or no problem with self-discipline, you may find it easy to exercise alone. But if you are like most people, you need a little help from your friends — which is why I recommend exercise classes. Chances are that you will follow through when you commit your time and money to an exercise instructor. You can boost your incentive by getting a friend to sign up, too.

I have also discovered that the time of day is another critical factor to take into account when setting up an exercise regimen. My personal choice is from 6 to 7 a.m. The early morning activity clears out the cobwebs in my brain and sets me up for a good, active day. If I don't do it at that time, procrastination wins out, and by the end of the day, guess what? I usually find I have managed to avoid exercising completely.

You may not be a morning person, so adjust accordingly. Just remember to be consistent and keep working at it until you find the right form of exercise and the right time to exercise.

NO MORE LAME EXCUSES

Remember how your subconscious tries to sabotage any new ideas you try to incorporate? This may also happen with your exercise program. You might go along with it for as much as a week or two, doing just fine, feeling ever so proud of yourself. Then you start finding excuses not to exercise: it's too cold today, there's not enough time, your jogging shorts are dirty, and on, and on. This is the time when it is vitally important to overcome all obstacles and go forth.

When you set the pattern on a consistent basis, you will eliminate those stupid excuses and be *eager* to exercise. I promise it will happen if you are consistent.

EXERCISE SATIATES YOUR APPETITE

Some clients tell me they are afraid to exercise because it may increase their appetites. This is a myth. When a person exercises, the hypothalamus, a part of the brain which controls the appetite, is stimulated. It responds by making the appetite seem quite satisfied.

A client of mine named Julia had a hard time accepting this. She proved it to herself when she joined a health spa. She worked out vigorously three days a week on her lunch break. She was surprised to discover she was thirsty, not hungry, after exercising. A glass of fruit juice became a very satisfying lunch on those three days a week. She was hungry and ready to eat lunch on the days she did not exercise. Julia was able to lose weight easily and painlessly, simply by introducing exercise into her life.

EXERCISE MELTS THE FAT

You get rid of fat and develop muscle in your body when you exercise. Muscle weighs more than fat, so don't be alarmed if that beautiful, smooth muscle running down your leg may be heavier than all the fat you have shed in the past month. Muscle tissue is compressed, firm, and takes up less space. You may not show a big difference in weight but you will notice a drop in your clothing size because your body is trimmer.

A PANACEA FOR MANY WOES

Many people consider exercise a grim treatment which must be endured in order to burn off calories. Actually, though, the greatest reward for working out is what it does for our *mental* health. Studies have shown exercise is the simplest way to relieve depression. Exercise helps you to feel good about yourself. Scientists are finding evidence that many chemical changes go on in the brain during physical activity, which is probably why many people report feeling very good about themselves after exercise. They can't explain why or how — it just happens, even though none of their outside problems have changed.

Tension and stress are kept at bay by a good exercise program. When you don't feel depressed, tense, or bad about yourself, chances are good you won't eat compulsively. Another very good thing about exercise is the fact that it releases toxins from your body — toxins which impair your health, damage your skin, and rob you of your energy.

EXERCISE ENCOURAGEMENT

Here are some affirmations which will help you to get into the proper frame of mind:

1. I always have the time, energy, and desire to exercise.

2. I now enjoy exercising.

3. It is now easy for me to follow my exercise plan on a consistent basis.

4. I now attract the right form of exercise into my life.

5. My body loves exercise!

6. My mind loves exercise!

7. My attitude toward exercise is now positive.

8. Exercise is fun and pleasurable.

9. Exercise is a pleasurable experience for me.

10. I now release any thoughts which have kept me from exercising in the past.

11. I now exercise regularly, and my body responds by giving me good health.

12. Exercise is an important pleasure that I give myself.

REMINDERS FROM CHAPTER SEVEN

1. Find a form of exercise that is fun!

2. Make it fit your time schedule, your skills, and your needs.

3. Analyze your excuses in order to find out what your resistance is.

4. Be consistent!

5. Exercise does positive things for both your body and your mind. It helps subdue your appetite, regulate your metabolism, release tension, burn fat, strengthen muscles, and much more.

8

BECOMING YOUR OWN THERAPIST

If you can find a competent therapist and/or a support group to help you in your quest, do it. Chances are, however, you may have to become your own therapist. This chapter contains guidelines for assessing your present lifestyle and incorporating some beneficial changes.

HONESTY IS THE BEST POLICY

Be honest with yourself as you answer the following questions, even if the truth is not palatable. Take heart if you don't feel like an overnight success. Exploring yourself can be painful, even though your efforts are rewarded with sweet freedom.

We humans have a built-in safety valve when faced with pain or frustration: we go "unconscious," becoming oblivious to the painful or frustrating stimulation. You will probably go unconscious or tune out as much as 80 percent of the material the first time you read this book, which is why I recommend you reread it, several times if necessary, until you have made the positive changes you want to make. Go over and over the questions and your answers in this chapter. Each time you repeat this process, you will learn something new about yourself which you may have not been ready to accept before.

1. Your weight history:

Check the box which corresponds to your weight and age in the chart below.

WEIGHT	AGE											
	10-12	13-14	15-17	18-20	21-25	26-30	31-35	36-40	41-45	46-50	51-55	56-60
300 & over												
290-299												
280-289												
270-279												
260-269												
250-259												
240-249												
230-239												
220-229												
210-219												
200-209												
190-199												
180-189												
170-179												
160-169												
150-159												
140-149												
130-139												
120-129												
110-119												
100-109												
90-99												

2. Using the preceding chart, list any changes, incidents, and feelings which took place whenever you gained a significant amount of weight.

AGE	SUMMARY OF EXPERIENCE
A.	
B.	
C.	
D.	
E.	
F.	
G.	
H.	

3. Now make a similar list detailing the times you lost weight.

AGE	SUMMARY OF EXPERIENCE
A.	
B.	
C.	
D.	
E.	
F.	
G.	

This exercise will enable you to see if there is a behavior pattern common to your weight gains and losses. For example, perhaps you tend to gain weight whenever you start a new romance. You should ask yourself what there is about falling in love and/or being single that makes you want to eat and gain weight. When you find the answer, you will have gained new power over your unconscious actions. You should then compose affirmations to correct your destructive thoughts.

4. List some of the other important goals in your life besides losing weight.

GOAL	VERY IMPORTANT	SOMEWHAT IMPORTANT	NOT IMPORTANT
Good health	☐	☐	☐
Satisfying sex	☐	☐	☐
Peace of mind	☐	☐	☐
Physical energy	☐	☐	☐
Academic success	☐	☐	☐
Career fulfillment	☐	☐	☐
Friends	☐	☐	☐
Recreation	☐	☐	☐
Financial prosperity	☐	☐	☐
Children	☐	☐	☐
Other_____	☐	☐	☐
_____	☐	☐	☐
_____	☐	☐	☐
_____	☐	☐	☐

As you analyze your responses to your life goals (other than losing weight), you will begin to get a clearer picture of your total personality. This is important because successful weight loss is not a one-dimensional phenomenon. You must consider yourself a total person, and give attention to all the facets of your life. This analysis may pinpoint an important part of your psyche which has been neglected because you have been preoccupied with losing weight.

5. Check which emotions and situations seem to trigger a response that makes you feel compelled to eat.

- ☐ Rejection
- ☐ Depression
- ☐ Failure
- ☐ Success
- ☐ Jealousy
- ☐ Loneliness
- ☐ Criticism
- ☐ Feeling inferior
- ☐ Boredom
- ☐ Cooking for others
- ☐ Fatigue

- ☐ Sexual problems
- ☐ Sexual pleasure
- ☐ Reading
- ☐ Making decisions
- ☐ Watching television
- ☐ Social situations
- ☐ Inclement weather
- ☐ Desire to avoid something
- ☐ Other (add any of your own)

This exercise makes you more aware of unconscious eating habits, and also gives you good material for creating effective affirmations to overcome your eating problem. For example, if you find making decisions difficult, you could create an affirmation like, "I now make decisions easily without eating."

Filling out the following four lists helps you to further identify previously undetected tendencies. You gain power over your eating habits simply by bringing these up to the conscious level. You can develop winning strategies as these realizations become more clear by using affirmations, visualizations, and any other form of self-help.

6. How I put myself in second place:

A.

B.

C.

D.

E.

7. Being overweight communicates the following statements to my mother, my father, my siblings, and my partner:

A.

B.

C.

D.

E.

8. What my parents have said about food, my body, and overweight people:

A.

B.

C.

D.

E.

9. The reasons I want to be thin:

A.

B.

C.

D.

E.

10. The last time I was at my perfect weight of _____ pounds was _____ . Write down how you felt about this time in your life, what was going on with your career, relationship, and health. What can you learn about the circumstances under which you gained weight?

11. On a separate piece of paper — or in the back of this book — chart your daily food habits for at least one week. Much of our eating is carried out on a subconscious level; this chart will enable you to become more conscious of your eating habits.

A. List the kinds and amounts of food you ate.

B. Where and when did you eat? (List the time of day or night.)

C. Was it a satisfaction or seduction food?

D. If you ate a seduction food, what were the precipitating circumstances, feelings and thoughts?

E. If you ate a satisfaction food, were you truly satisfied?

12. On a separate piece of paper, make a list of things you do to boost your self-esteem. Here are some suggestions:

A. Do affirmations for improving self-esteem. This is the best way to tune into your capacity for self-love.

B. Take each mistake as an opportunity to grow and understand yourself. Don't beat yourself up for your human frailties.

C. Learn to accept compliments and acknowledge-ments. Simply say, "Thank you." You don't need to return the compliments, just accept them.

D. Reward yourself with something nice other than food. Give your body an occasional treat, such as a massage, pedicure, or facial.

E. Keep a success diary for a few days so you can record all your big and little successes.

F. Take yourself out to dinner. Don't just grab a ham-burger to go and eat it in your car. Make reservations at your favorite restaurant. Go alone and acknowledge to yourself that you are alone because you like your own company. Don't take papers from the office or a magazine to keep yourself occupied. Order what you really want and enjoy yourself.

G. Express your self-love while looking in the mirror. Choose one part of your body that you really appre-ciate. Even if it is only your earlobes, you should study and compliment it. Choose a new part each day, until your whole body gets attention.

H. Send yourself cards and letters. Pick a pretty card and write yourself a loving note. Address, stamp, and mail it. It is a wonderful affirmation of your self-love when you receive it.

I. Do work you love. If you hate your job, you must find a way to give it up. I realize you can't rush out and give up your meal ticket right away. But you must change it soon if it is not good for you. The situations you put yourself in each day are a reflection of your own self-worth.

J. Hang a picture of yourself on the wall.

K. Take a bath by candlelight while you listen to self-esteem affirmations in the background.

L. Spend a day in bed. You don't have to sleep; just lay around and rest, read, paint your nails, and coddle yourself.

The suggestions above are models for building up your self-esteem. They are all pleasant, though you may be a bit skittish about some of them, simply because you have never tried them before. Give them a chance (or three) and you will soon reap the positive rewards. Have fun!

13. Visualizations: The best way to do this exercise is to record it on a cassette tape. First, read the instructions slowly, preferably taping the visualization you want to do. Then lie down, close your eyes, listen to your cassette tape, and follow the visualization. Try to be aware of your reactions to the different visualizations and use this newly acquired information to gain more knowledge about yourself.

I have provided three visualization exercises for you to try — however, you will probably discover that the most effective exercises for you are the ones you create yourself. My work with women of all ages and personalities has repeatedly proven that each person has her own unique reaction to the exercises. For example, in one of my exercises I have a client visualize putting her most negative thoughts into a brown paper bag. She then places this bag into a fireplace and lights it. Her negative thoughts go up in flames and out the chimney, never to return again.

One client uses this method several times a day, and finds that it continues to be valuable for her, day after day. Another woman said she couldn't possibly carry out this visualization exercise with a straight face. It was the most ridiculous thing she had ever heard of.

Use your imagination to create the appropriate visualization for you. Here are three possibilities — remember that it is most effective to use just one visualization at a time.

A. Imagine that you are standing on a bridge which spans a huge river. You stand on the bridge with a big gunny sack in your hand. Imagine you are stuffing all your old negative ideas about losing weight into the sack. Put in negative statements such as, "Losing weight is hard for me," "I have to deprive myself of food to lose extra weight," "My body will always be fat and ugly," and "I need my extra weight to be safe." You are also depositing all your frustrations, anger, disgust, failures, and hate into this sack.

Now the bag is full; take a strong rope and close the bag, tying it securely. Watch yourself toss the bag over the side of the bridge. Away it goes, into the water, down the rapids, far away from you, never to return. As the bag with your negativity disappears, you notice a beautiful, vibrant rainbow forming over the river. Each of the rainbow's hues represents a new, positive feeling you have about yourself. The pink is your emerging self-love; violet is your personal power; gold is your self-determination; blue is your peace and tranquility; green represents joy and self-confidence. Take a few moments to let these positive feelings become a part of you. When you are ready, open your eyes.

B. Imagine you are looking at yourself in a full-length mirror. See yourself as you are today. Then imagine for a moment that your hands have magical power: as you run your hands over your body, the excess pounds and inches disappear.

You now see your body exactly as you want it to be. Now imagine your body without any clothes. Admire your side profile, then your back, and finally your front. Now imagine your perfect body with clothing on — the kind of clothes you love to wear. As you now look at yourself in the mirror, do you feel safe, happy, and powerful? Or do you feel frightened and weak? What other feelings emerge when you visualize yourself at your perfect weight?

Watch yourself stand on a set of scales; you are at your perfect weight. This is how you see yourself, always; this is always how you think about yourself. Now, let a peaceful calm fill your mind and body. When you are ready, open your eyes.

C. You are sitting in front of a fireplace, with a warm, crackling fire. Your mind and body are permeated with warmth and coziness. You are cracking walnuts from a nearby basket. Each time you crack a walnut, you find it contains a piece of paper. Each paper contains the answer to one of your questions about your "weight problem."

Your first question is to determine your greatest obstacle when it comes to losing weight. Now crack a walnut and read what is on the paper to find the answer to your question. Now you can crack open as many as you wish and find whatever answers you need. When you are ready, you may open your eyes.

14. Write a list of all the pleasant things you can do for yourself whenever you are tempted to eat seducer foods. Keep the list handy so you can substitute one of these things for the seducer food. I'll start the list for you; I want you to add to it, however.

A. Take a bubble bath.
B. Go for a walk.
C. See a movie
D. Call a friend (splurge on long distance).
E. Give yourself a manicure.
F. Get a massage.
G. Take a nap.
H. Indulge yourself by reading a schmaltzy novel.
I. Put on some boogie music and dance.
J. _____
K. _____
L. _____
M. _____
N. _____
O. _____

GIVE YOURSELF THE BEST — YOU DESERVE IT!

Provide yourself with all the self-help material you can find. Use cassette tapes to continue learning and to keep up your motivation(an order form is in the back of the book). Schedule time on your appointment calendar exclusively devoted to self-therapy. Consistency and self-belief does pay off.

REMINDERS FROM CHAPTER EIGHT

1. Seek a competent therapist and/or a support group if possible.

2. Be willing to be honest with yourself.

3. Repeat the processes in this chapter over and over, until you understand yourself.

4. Provide yourself with all the self-help material you can find.

5. Read and re-read this entire book.

9

REMINDERS

Here is a list of reminders and suggestions to insure your success. If you ever feel discouraged, just check this list and see what you can do to stir up your enthusiasm.

1. Visualize yourself at your perfect weight and size.

2. Make a treasure map.

3. Keep a journal of your feelings and experiences with food and your body. This is a good mode of self-expression.

4. Practice visualization exercises. These are positive tools for changing your negative beliefs to positive. They also help relieve stress and tension.

5. Examine the foods you eat. Determine if you are eating seduction or satisfaction foods.

6. Practice your affirmation exercises consistently.

7. Enroll in an assertiveness training class.

8. Find a form of exercise and do it on a regular basis.

9. Read and reread this book.

ABOUT THE AUTHOR

KAREN DARLING is a counselor in private practice who lectures widely and conducts seminars on weight control, eating disorders, and developing self-esteem. She is a consultant to physicians and psychologists on permanent weight-loss methods, as well as a teacher on the college level.

Ms. Darling appears regularly on radio and television programs to discuss her work. She is a former professional model who produced and hosted her own daily television and radio shows for seven years.

She is a committed activist, and lobbies on behalf of world peace and environmental and women's issues. She lives with her daughter and a menagerie of domestic and wild animals on a farm in Ashland, Oregon.

KAREN DARLING'S WORKSHOPS

Karen Darling presents lectures and workshops for groups anywhere in the world. A program can be tailor-made to fit the needs of your group or organization.

Karen is dedicated to the understanding of weight problems, and she is constantly seeking new and helpful ideas to add to her program. For more information on workshops and lectures, write to Karen Darling, P.O. Box 915, Ashland, Oregon 97520.